Parenting
a Child with
Crohn's Disease

RACHEL M. COOPER

Fulton Books, Inc.
Meadville, PA

Published by Fulton Books 2021

ISBN 978-1-63860-486-0 (paperback)
ISBN 978-1-63860-487-7 (digital)

Printed in the United States of America

CHAPTER 1

What Is Crohn's Disease

Parenting a child with Crohn's disease or inflammatory bowel disease has been a challenge from day one. IBD is a broad term that is used to describe disorders that involve chronic inflammation in the digestive tract. I didn't know what Crohn's disease was until my son's gastroenterologist specialist told me to research it in order to become more familiar with Crohn's. What I found out is there are different forms of inflammatory bowel diseases (IBD) on two levels. There are many but I'm more familiar with ulcerative colitis and Crohn's disease which my son, Cj, was diagnosed with at an early age. Ulcerative colitis is a chronic inflammatory bowel disease that causes inflammation in the digestive tract and mainly shows up in the colon itself. Crohn's disease is also a chronic inflammatory bowel disease that affects the lining of the digestive tract and can show up in any area from the mouth to the anus. Each person who is affected by either disease may have different experiences in symptoms and may take different medications, depending on the severity of their case. Each case is different because some people who are diagnosed with IBD may have light, mild, or severe symptoms, depending on the individual.

Having this disease should be taken seriously, no matter how you look at it. Paying close attention to your body and what's going on with it can help you in the long run and deal with Crohn's disease in an effective way. Cj was diagnosed with Crohn's, back in the year of 2001 at age seven. He is now twenty-six years of age and still managing it as a normal part of his daily routine. Everything started when Cj was losing weight drastically in a two-month span. Cj was a healthy, nine pounds and six ounces baby boy, who myself and family never thought Crohn's disease would play a major part in his life. I remember age seven like it was yesterday because Cj was a very articulate young man, who mapped out his college career at this exact age. There was a map on his bedroom wall of all the steps he needed to take in order to fulfill his dream of attending college after high school. What was shocking, Cj wasn't even in the fifth grade, and he had determination for college life at an early age. Quite impressive as I look back!

As I seen him lose weight at first stage of Crohn's, embarking on his life, I told myself maybe he had the stomach flu. And it will end in a week or so. From day to day, his weight continued to disappear in a rapid manner, and after a week, his regular doctor saw him and concluded that it was the stomach flu, which will leave soon. The doctor stated, with plenty of fluids and rest, Cj should jump back to normal in no time. Not only did I notice weight loss but also frequent visits to the bathroom. Everything he ate it went straight through him as though he was cleansing himself with no help of pills, certain cleansing diets, or those horrible quick fix tonics. After three weeks, I began to worry because the flu doesn't last that long, especially with children who is healthy. There were doctor visits in between on testing to see what was going on with Cj's body. After four weeks, the weight was still disappearing, and Cj looked malnourished and weak to the point where he could barely walk.

Finally, I received a call from Stanford Children Hospital that an appointment was setup with a gastroenterologist specialist that heard about Cj's situation, which they wanted to see him immediately. At this point, Cj had lost so much weight. His life would have ended if it wasn't for the specialist, jumping right into action on giving him full doses of liquid steroids called prednisone. Yes, I said prednisone. The wonder drug that help heals quickly the problem areas inside the body. But has side effects, which weaken bones and stun children's growth if taken consistently over a long period of time. At this point, he was in the hospital for a month's stay and was treated as a special patient with a serious condition. Only few parents really knew what Crohn's disease was because there were few cases back in 2001.

The symptoms that Cj experienced was fatigue, cramping in abdomen, pain on left side of stomach, fevers, weight loss, frequent diarrhea, loss of appetite, and rectal bleeding. As you may guess, this was the severe aspect of Crohn's disease at it's all time high. As Cj became better while in hospital, he started to pick up his weight, and his appetite came back with a vengeance. He wanted to eat everything and was hungry all the time, which is what prednisone does to your system when taking as a medication. I was very happy to have my son back at his normal self. The prednisone steroids healed him to recovery, and we were going back home to our comfortable lives again. Or so I thought it would be comfortable or even back to normal.

I can remember I had taken off work for many days during the time Cj was admitted into hospital. This is just the beginning of what is to come when Crohn's disease takes a role in your child's life or someone you know. There will be many more hospital stays and doctor visits, depending on the severity of the disease. I say, arm yourself with knowledge of every aspect of Crohn's. I have learned a lot and continue to learn more as time goes on. I felt as though I was being cursed for something I did, but why did Cj have to pay the price of being sick from day to day. He couldn't play like the other kids in the neighborhood because his energy level was always down. He asked questions as to why he was diagnosed with Crohn's, and will he become normal at some point.

My suggestion to all parents is to keep the line of communication open, along with an open mind. As a parent, the more you learn about Crohn's, the more the condition becomes bearable and easy to deal with in your household. I was very curious and willing to learn what I needed to know in case Cj had questions and thoughts about the disease. To some degree or another, I sensed that Cj became interested in what he had rather than shying away from it. Because he saw me as his mom interested in wanting to know what he was diagnosed with and trying to figure things out. When a child sees the parent learning all there is to know, they tend to deal with the disease on a level that establishes a more positive attitude about what they are dealing with.

CHAPTER 2

The Effect Crohn's Have On You and Your Child

The effect Crohn's disease can have on you and your child can be from anywhere to stressful and irritability with exhaustion added to infinity. When I say there were days I wanted to pull my hair out and bite a few people that was irritating to me or making the situation worse, I probably would have if I didn't have Christ in my life. The reason Crohn's take a toll on a person is because we don't think that it is possible for our child to get the diagnosis in the first place. We, as the parents, can't wrap our heads around the thought of Crohn's becoming our reality or any disease for that matter. If we are real with ourselves, we also know that things happen to people at all stages of life, but we just don't believe it can happen to us or our children. This is a normal feeling but also realize the world we live in. There is a whole world out there which is recognizable by the billion-dollar-a year pharmaceutical industry that creates tons of medications for all types of illnesses and diseases we have never heard of until it hits us right in the face and inside our homes.

After Cj was diagnosed, he became better and back to somewhat normal. I learned quickly after his release from hospital, four to five months had passed, he started losing weight again. I assumed he was cured because the specialist that nursed him back to health didn't explain he needed to always be on medication with Crohn's for the rest of his life. No conversation about the disease, after going home, was even brought up when being released from hospital. I became stressed and irritable and angry because I couldn't figure out what was going on.

I ended up seeing the same pattern when Cj became very ill from previous admission to hospital. I was alert, and so I researched all gastroenterologist specialists in the Bay Area. I found one and had good vibes after reading what their credentials were and the specialty at hand. I called to make an appointment, and to my satisfaction, this was the beginning of a new life it had felt like. To my surprise, when meeting the new pediatric gastroenterologist specialist, he told me that I should take time to research what Crohn's disease is and that Cj will need to be on medication for the rest of his life. He explained to me what the word *chronic* meant because that is exactly what Cj had, a chronic disease. I was a little shocked because I didn't have knowledge of this information, and I was wondering why the other specialist who saw him early on didn't relay this information to me.

I became very happy and excited with this specialist because he had informed me of what will be expected and what I needed to do as a parent. I even told myself that I witnessed a doctor who really cared about my son and his other patients he may have seen for same conditions. This was the beginning of a beautiful doctor, patient, and parent friendship I seen. This alone released a lot of pressure off me because now I had somebody in my corner to help me and Cj fight this ugly and disrespectful monster called Crohn's. Most doctors have that *god* complex like they know it all but not this specialist. He immediately informed me that what a mom wants to do then he will follow her lead. He kept me up-to-date on all decisions and ideas he came up with. If I gave him the go ahead with what he felt could help Cj, I became free from any worries.

This is the type of specialist that any parent could want or wish for because he isn't hardnosed to the fact that he will try anything and everything on your child. He wants your input at every stage of getting to the point where your child is in remission or at least feeling better. Another thing which helped me deal with this monster is this chronic disease was forever. Chronic means ongoing, and this was another word I learned. Sure, I've heard of the word *chronic* before but never had to completely understand it. As I read more on Crohn's, I began to stress less and less! If you are not on the same page as specialist and that specialist keep you in the dark about things on what they are going to do or what future plans are, this can have a negative effect on you and your child. I tell you right now, you will become more worried. You will also experience issues within yourself such as eating unhealthy and sleeplessness at certain times. You have to stay healthy for your child and create instances where you plan for each day. This is easier because you stay ahead of what is needed on your part as a parent.

I suggest you inform your boss or supervisor on this matter with your child as soon as the diagnosis is given. There is a way to take precautions for missing work when your child has a slew of appointments with doctors and specialist, along with blood test. I say blood test because with Crohn's, a plethora of test will be needed in order to keep up with body functions. Functions such as the heart, liver, kidneys, and growth are very much important when taking medications. At work, I signed up for FMLA which is the Family Medical Leave Act. Having FMLA covers you at work when you're not there. You get to take paid leave for medical and family reasons with a continuation of group health insurance coverage under the same terms and conditions, as if you did not take leave from work. You get twelve work weeks of leave in a twelve-month period, which makes it easier on parents being away from work. You may not have to take all the days consistently. I took hours instead of days intermittently, which kept me from using up all the time I needed. Either I would go to work late or be there early and leave for the rest of the day, depending on Cj's appointments.

My son had to have blood test drawn a week before his specialist's appointment, in order for his specialist to know the results in what was going on with Cj. Seeing that his condition was severe, he was taking blood test sometimes twice a week and seeing the specialist twice a week. The specialist's main concern was if medications were interfering with Cj's body organs like his liver, if white blood cell count was low or high, if there was inflammation and how much, and if his sed rate was high.

Most of these tests were inflammatory marker test called CRP and ESR. CRP test measures the level of one specific protein called acute phase protein. Meaning it increases when a person has certain diseases that causes inflammation. ESR are tests that measures many different types of protein where the red blood cells fall to bottom of tube, leaving plasma at the top. The rate which red blood cells separate from the plasma at the top with high ESR indicates a high rate of inflammation. Don't worry if you are not up-to-date with all tests because you will learn as you go. I suggest asking the specialist for a copy of the test results because you can familiarize yourself with words on the test that will mean a great deal. If you do this as a parent, you will be able to relate on what the specialist is talking about. The more you know, the less stress you will become.

Medications

Being diagnosed with Crohn's disease also brings the world of medication. The goal of Crohn's disease is remission, few, or no symptoms. Every two years, a new medication is being created for Crohn's. There are different medications given for different reasons, and time will tell if they are working or not. There are antibiotics when infections occur, Aminosalicylates (5-ASA's) given orally or rectally to decrease inflammation, corticosteroids given to reduce inflammation by suppressing the immune system to help with moderate to severe Crohn's symptoms, immune modifiers given so inflammation doesn't continue, and biologic therapies given to reduce inflammation by targeting a specific pathway and is normally given to patients who has not responded to conventional medications.

There are two major worlds medication revolve around. There are medications that the FDA approves which is said to be safe for humans, and there are medications which become experimental when nothing else works. Crohn's medications are for controlling the inflammation that may be causing most of your symptoms. My son has taken 6MP, prednisone, Humira, Flagyl, methotrexate, and Entyvio along with some antibiotics when needed. Most are in pill form, but the Crohn's medication itself is normally given by injections or intravenously at an infusion clinic.

Cj's Entyvio can take forty-five minutes to a few hours to be given, depending on whether or not the nurse can find his vein immediately at time of distribution. The Humira would take three to four hours, depending on dosage by doctor. When a medication stops working for Crohn's, it is easy to start noticing the signs. Cj will start gradually losing his appetite, slowly start dropping weight, and I see there was more frequent stops to the bathroom. This means that inflammation starts building up in his digestive tract, and also the signs alerting me it's time for another specialist visit to get a jump on the disease. The medication stops working because his body started producing antibodies which will start rejecting the medication. Dealing with the conventional meds Cj was his specialist's worst case because he would only respond to meds for maybe two and three months at a time. Humira was the first medication for Crohn's that seemed to work for about five years.

Hopefully as time goes on, new medications will be made to combat this disease and become less harmful in which we see more of a remission phase. If it wasn't for medications, things would be a bit more complicated. But I choose to think positive and feel blessed to know that scientists out there are doing their part in saving lives.

CHAPTER 4

Complications

The complications that arise with Crohn's disease are anemia, rejection of medication, weak bones, slow growth, and infections that could turn deadly if not treated early. Anemia comes when the red blood cells are low due to medications lowering the immune system with my son's case. Cj became anemic and was put on a certain dosage of ferrous sulfate (iron). Rejection of medications is not good when there is many that has been tried by a child or individual with Crohn's. Cj has rejected many medications to the point where we were thinking about trying experimental medications. It was a blessing for new meds to come out at the right time. Cj joints inside. His body became weak at times due to prednisone intake over long periods of time. Most doctors don't like for children to take steroids over a long-time frame because of weak bones and stunned growth. Knowing my son's situation, I actually think he did well on steroids, seeing that his condition was highly severe.

What I loved about his pediatrician gastro specialist is that he monitored every medication especially the steroids. He would gradually prescribe my son prednisone at small dosages at a time and build up to more if needed. He then would keep him on it for three to four months only, and at the end of the fourth month, he would start weaning him off the steroid. What I learned is that you can't just quit taking steroids, cold turkey, or there are serious withdrawals. The complications with steroids are headaches and a sense of upset moments with an angry attitude, which I noticed when Cj was on steroids, and also drastic weight gain at a fast rate. I didn't care about the weight gain as much because my son needed weight on his body, which I thought it can help aid his body to fight Crohn's more effectively.

Another complication would be intravenous meds can seem hectic for the simple fact some patients have smaller veins. This can become a problem if nurses aren't used to finding small veins. Cj have small veins, and they become smaller if he happens to be dehydrated, haven't been consuming lots of liquids, or food that may have more liquids in them. One way to beat this issue is making sure your child or any individual drinks plenty of fluids the day before visiting infusion clinic. I have seen nurses plop a heated pack on the arm where they look for the vein, but honestly, this really didn't work for my son. After all the doctor appointments, emergency room, and hospital stays, I also learned nurses in the ER was more equipped in finding Cj's veins. Simply because they deal with more emergency situations than a regular nurse who only works on a certain ward in the hospital.

ER nurses become a specialist because of emergency, fast-paced, stressed moments where they have to think on their feet at all times. I actually love seeing a nurse who walks right in, introduces themselves while striking up a conversation with Cj, looks at his arm, and out of nowhere, cleans the area with alcohol swab; sticks the needle right in vein, looks up and smile while saying, "Okay, all done!" I mean those be the highlight of the blood draw appointments. Aside from the fact Cj questions nurses on why they decided to get into that field. Lots of nice moments when things may seem dark. I love it!

I advise all parents to pay attention to all complications that may arise because this will prepare you, in case it happens again. There can be many difficult days, but it will help you to be patient and stay focused on your child's situation with Crohn's. Those difficult moments will turn into happy ones when the time comes. From my experience, difficult moments only mean you will work through whatever is necessary while creating a path to wellness for your child or family member who suffers from Crohn's Disease.

This new virus called Novel Coronavirus (COVID-19) is a death threat to any individual who has Crohn's or any other inflammatory bowel disease. I say death threat because most of the medications for controlling Crohn's will lower your immune system. It's like when you're sitting up, watching TV, and that unwanted commercial come on about the disease or illness a person might have. First, they talk about the illness or problem and then how good the medication works. Then dive right into the side effects in how it causes damage to your body organs while including the fact it may cause death. I mean really! Who wants to take a medication that may kill them if they're trying to live by helping their illness in the first place? When I first heard of this virus and how fast it was taking lives, I immediately grabbed my stomach and said to myself, "What the hell is going on!"

And also "Cj is about to be on lockdown like an inmate on death row." All I could think of is this virus is gonna be my worst nightmare ever, especially with Cj having a precondition already! As days went by, I came to the conclusion that I was doing most of the tasks already, like using hand sanitizer, washing my hands frequently, sterilizing door knobs and handles, wiping everything down in my home, spraying Lysol in my household daily to keep bacteria and viruses from spreading, and making sure Cj is living in a healthy safe environment. I have my mom to thank for instilling in me the reality of my childhood, where she made me and my sisters clean at a young age. Yes, we had household chores every day after school. Soon as we step our foot in the front door, we completed our chores whether it was washing dishes, cleaning the bathroom, or straightening up and vacuuming the living room floor. After, we would find a quiet place and complete our homework. If something was left undone, we would definitely hear about it.

I remember one night I forgot to wash dishes and called myself going to bed early, being tired from school and the morning rush of waking up all week. I was not a morning person and still not till this day. I was sleeping so good and even was dreaming I had started college. I was walking on Stanford University campus, smiling, and taking in the beautiful vibes of how the old buildings look. I was far in my dream and all of a sudden, I heard my mom calling me. I'm thought to myself, *why am I hearing my mom voice on campus?* Slowly, it became very loud. And then it hit me, I was not at Stanford, and I better wake up real fast because my mom was not yelling for nothing. I jumped out of my bed to look and see what time it was. I looked at the clock, and it said 3:30 a.m. Trying to figure out what she wanted, I walked in the kitchen where I heard her voice and then it all came to me. Dang it! I forgot to wash the dishes before I went to bed! Oh no! Her next words were, "If you don't get in here and wash these dishes, it will get ugly!"

I was so mad and tired, I just decided not to put up a fuss and get the dishes out the way. I knew going forward I will not ever forget to complete my chores before going to bed. I learned two valuable lessons that morning. Do not go to bed before completing my chores, and stop staying up all week late on school nights so I won't be tired. Long story short, me and my sisters have OCD when it comes to cleanliness, so we have some experience on this new virus. Now that COVID-19 has become a part of the world's everyday life, I would say I was practicing cleanliness for years. I work from home since March of 2020, and I am very thankful for being allowed to do this while our government try to get a handle on this deadly virus. I don't think anyone would have seen this virus coming by a long shot.

Even though I care about the next person during this hectic time, I cannot understand why people are buying up all the toilet paper. I mean if I didn't know any better, I would think we had a shortage on this item. And even more so, why would I hoard tissue from others? Talk about tissue crisis. People, please get a grip! Be respectful of other lives and leave some tissues for a neighbor or friend. I can be nosey at times, and I am not afraid to admit it. But what I have also noticed is the tissue and paper towel aisle in every store was bare, like the bottom of my feet. Why is the soap aisle still full? This is the aisle that should be wiped clean. I'm not saying we should fight over soap, but I would expect it to be a few arguments and disputes for the time being. When I think about this COVID-19, I ponder in deep thought. Because whereas I was able to buy Lysol and other products, now it's a shortage due to others being afraid and greediness. I understand that we are afraid of this virus, but some people just don't realize there are others who need these products in order to live, especially if they have diseases and illnesses. Like myself, I was using these products before the COVID-19 made its appearance. Now, I can't find a can of Lysol in any store. It's scary because I don't want to go grocery shopping and come back with COVID-19 when Cj lives with me. That would not be pretty!

I don't know anyone close to me who have lost their lives due to contracting COVID-19, and I would like to keep it that way! However, my heart goes out to all families who have lost a loved one! I know it could be a hard thing, losing someone. I am concerned about our older generation and people who have illnesses which would be compromised due to this virus like Cj. Lately as the months passed by, COVID-19 has been attacking all ages. Senior citizens, teenagers, young children of ages five to twelve, and now college students. I say arm yourselves with building up your immune system with vitamins and minerals and not with toilet paper. Cj and I take regular dosages of vitamins plus extra vitamin C and D with zinc daily. We drink lots of water to keep our bodies hydrated. Because I am older, I drink a lemon tonic made up of hot water, over a sliced whole lemon, and let steep for fifteen minutes. This may not work for everyone, but it helps me. I was taught growing up that lemons are a wonder fruit, and I intend to keep this as my ritual drink as long as I live. I wish everyone well, even the maniac shoppers. Please be safe, people.

Special Diets and Certain Foods

It's a good idea to ask your child's doctor about taking supplements. Because it helps if their eating pattern is down, in which their body isn't getting the right amount of nutrients especially if they are vomiting and having a bad case of diarrhea due to symptoms with Crohn's. My son didn't have a special diet because he was and still is a picky eater. And his doctor informed us that he can eat anything at this stage just to get food inside his system. As Cj's mother, I had to step in and monitor what he ate. Because if he is having issues with his digestive tract, I had to scan foods that I felt would do more harm than good. For instance, I didn't think popcorn, nuts, corn, or anything with a hull on it were suitable for his Crohn's. Seeing that the digestive tract from a normal human have issues of breaking down these types of food, Cj had to be careful. A Crohn's patient, I think, would definitely cause harsh issues in the digestive tract in consuming these foods mentioned earlier, but for every case, things can be quite different. I have a friend who was diagnosed with Crohn's about three years ago at age forty-three. From my knowledge, she doesn't have a special diet because I've seen her eat everything under the sun. Her case was different from my son's case because she had more inflammation issues than losing weight or taking many trips to the bathroom which my son had.

I suggest parents to pay close attention to eating patterns whereas some foods can cause more problems than necessary, or trigger complications within Crohn's. Gastric episodes can also come from foods high in fiber. Be aware of spicy foods, this caused my son to endure a lot of flatulence (farting) on certain days. Eating at a certain time, more on the early side, can help with bedtime issues. All the talk about GMO (genetically modified organisms) should be looked at also. I can't wrap my head around this GMO crap, but I take each day at a time. When Cj was diagnosed, myself finding out what was good and what was bad meant. I was at war. Certain foods can be good in a bad way and bad in a good way. Eating something bad in moderation cannot harm you if you're eating good foods also.

I stopped buying regular cow milk because it made our stomach turn into knots, and I found that it carried bacteria in it, even after it was processed. The bacteria may not harm a regular human, but I decided to leave it out of our diet. And I started buying almond and coconut milk for better digestion. We haven't had regular milk in over twenty years, and I'm proud to say that I do not miss it. I'll say that I cook with it here and there in small amounts. It doesn't affect us as if we drank it from a glass. I buy brown organic eggs and most of my fruits and veggies are the same. Because what grows from the ground or tree when eating it, you have to think about the skin that has either been sitting in dirt or on a tree that has been sprayed with chemicals.

Even if you wash the fruit or vegetable, that chemical, such as pesticides, has soaked into the skin, and now you're going to eat it. Like I said, this may not affect a normal person without any diseases, but I want to make the proper decision for Cj and give him the best when it comes to eating healthy for his situation. Cj do not need to add extra complications to his life just because he wanted to eat that regular apple with chemicals on it. I'm here to guide and discipline him for the times when he ends up living on his own. In that order!

Procedures and Surgeries

Over the years, Cj has had two major surgeries which I gladly thank his pediatric gastro specialist. You have some surgeons who get happy, and all they want to do is cut on a person. They remind me of a car salesman who will lower a person in his grasp, tell the person all they want to hear while leaving out the important details, then sale you the car. Only later to find out the car payment you talked about is $200 higher than the actually agreed upon amount. Now, he's lurking around a corner, looking at you from a distance, wondering at what moment will you find out that your car payment will be $500. Let's just call that car salesman what he really is—a shark out for blood!

Well, there are surgeons who do the same. They will give you all the reasons why getting surgery will help improve your life, and how you really need to do it. I'm very thankful that Cj's specialist stayed away from recommending him to get surgery at every incident, where things weren't looking okay. Getting surgery for a Crohn's patient should be the very last resort. The specialist didn't want Cj getting a lot of X-rays either. It does more harm to the body than we know.

Cj's first surgery was at age twenty-three, and it went well. The surgery was for him to receive an ileostomy, which is a small opening on the stomach to get rid of waste in a small bag because he no longer can use the bathroom in a normal way. This was supposed to be just for about three months and was reversible. Cj wasn't healing as he should. So it was discussed by the surgeon if Cj would want to keep the ileostomy in order to have a better quality of life, and be able to live somewhat of a normal but different way. To my surprise, Cj decided to keep it permanently because he didn't want to deal with his Crohn's any further. Besides, just to say if he would have had the operation to reverse everything back to normal, there could be the possibility of Crohn's showing back up in same area. And Cj would have had to repeat the same surgery when he already had been at that stage in the first place.

To be honest, I was nervous and scared at the thought of Cj wouldn't be able to function like everyone else. Now that I look back on it, Cj made the best decision he could for himself, and I am very proud of him. He adjusted to what he felt he had to do, and I was there to support him in any way I could. When his second surgery took place for the permanent ileostomy, he also had to get plastic surgery at the same time. Due to the anal needing muscle to be placed there, seeing it needed some type of tissue in order to heal properly. The plastic surgeon took his left ab from chest and placed it inside his anus, and this would complete all steps for a different positive outcome. The surgery was successful, and he is now in the healing stage. For the time being, there is no more running to restrooms, worrying about infection in problem area, and no more bleeding.

I remembered Cj's second emergency hospital stay. It was due to an infection that became really bad. He was in high school when I had to pull him out and put him in independent studies, where Cj went to school once a week because he was too sick to attend regular school. I remembered he stayed in the hospital for a month and two weeks. Let me just give you the tea! See what had happened was, his Crohn's area (anal) became infected so bad that his white blood cell count went to zero. If you don't know what this means, I'll tell you! When a person's white blood cell count goes to zero, this means that any bacteria, virus, or infection that gets inside the body will kill that person because they have no white blood cells to help immune system fight. I was happy he was in the hospital already at that time.

His specialist told me that he was scared, and he didn't know what else to do at this time. So in other words, he basically said there is a possibility my son may die. I can remember like this was yesterday. Cj's specialist talked to me outside the hospital room door by myself with no one around but me. I had a feeling that he was going to tell me something to this effect. Cj was hooked up to all kinds of tubes and thingamajigs. Slowly, he was slipping away. And after the specialist walked away, I just looked up into the ceiling, placed both my hands together, and prayed to God and asked him to heal my son. I thought if God worked his magic through these doctors, that they would be able to perform a miracle for CJ. Then, I would get my wonderful son back, and all would be amazing. After I prayed, fifteen minutes later, the specialist came back and told me he talked to a few of his colleagues. And they will come and take a look at CJ, so they would be able to come up with a solution. At this point, I crossed my fingers and looked into the air as if I was talking to God. And I said quietly, "Thank you, my Lord and Savior."

Now, I know he was about to do something great! The next day, I'm sitting there on the side of Cj's hospital bed, minding my own business, and here comes a doctor from out of nowhere. The doctor introduced himself as an infectious disease (ID) doctor who would come by to check up on Cj daily and run some test. I was excited, knowing there was another doctor also evaluating Cj's situation with infection. On same day, another doctor rolled inside the room, introducing himself as a blood specialist doctor. I knew exactly what type of doctor this was because I worked at VA Hospital for over ten years. This doctor was called a hematologist, who does the study of blood. This second doctor, who entered the room, relayed to us that he also would be checking on Cj for some days to come and run test.

I knew that the next few days would be crucial, due to the fact that Cj's specialist would not allow anyone in the room who had any symptoms of a cold, flu. Even fresh fruits, vegetables, and any plants as a gift, can enter. I'll say in a matter of twenty-four hours, Cj's specialist came back to visit in notifying us he wants to try a procedure to see if it will help save Cj's life. The specialist talked it over with me while Cj was weak and asleep. It was as if Cj was holding on to life as long as possible. Cj would see my face and perk up a bit, knowing I was at his bedside at all times. The nurses noticed the bond me and

Cj had while in the hospital. There was an effect we had on each other that no one else could understand but us. Sure, the nurses saw it and was amazed at our chemistry but didn't completely understand the deepness of our bond. A mother's love goes beyond what is necessary. The specialist said to me, "I want to give Cj some medicine by shooting it to his bones, where his bones can kick out white blood cells at a fast pace. But I worry it will go at a very fast rate, and his body may start attacking itself to where the procedure will not work."

I nodded my head as though I was agreeing for him to proceed. I said, "Okay!" I knew that if white blood cells were made, and the more the count goes up, this will give Cj a fighting chance. The specialist and I were on same page as always, but I had a feeling this would work. So I prayed again and asked God to take over to perform his miracle like I knew he could. The same day, nurses enter the room and started giving Cj the miracle medicine. I sat there with all the confidence in the world and became very calm. The next day came and I just finished breakfast. Cj was laying there with a little more energy than yesterday. The ID doctor came into the room and told us Cj didn't have any infectious disease so that made me smile like the Kool-Aid man. He said there is nothing to worry about, and as he started walking close to the front door to leave, he looked back and said he still will be checking on Cj daily.

The hematologist doctor came by twenty minutes later and also said Cj has no blood illnesses and from the test, speculation was ruled out. With hearing the good news for today, I think my happiness went to a level one hundred times infinity. I just said to myself, "Only God can work this kind of magic."

I then said, "Thank you, God. I see and feel you even though I don't see you." Cj started moving around in bed a little more, and I'm noticing his energy level is increasing. Cj's specialist (doctor amazing) comes in and tells me he has found that Cj has no other problems. And the only thing that made him sick was that his Crohn's was infected badly in the lower area of intestines. This was always the problem area from day one. He also told me Cj's test was coming back where his white blood cell count was growing. The procedure was working, and Cj was now out of the danger phase. Days go by and Cj become responsive and alert again. His appetite was back to normal, and he was smiling. After a month, we were going home, and life is wonderful! My job is not over yet because I have continued to pay close attention to everything more so than before. All I can say is, "The good, the bad, and the grateful!"

CHAPTER 7

Staying Ahead of Crohn's as a Parent

Each day, after your child is diagnosed with Crohn's, will be a challenge, and there will be tons of things you will learn as you go. Of course, you will make mistakes, assume the worse, and at some point, shut down due to being exhausted, feeling overwhelmed, and for the most part, not know what to do at times. This type of attitude is perfectly normal because we, as human beings, do not have all the answers. Even doctors and specialists will not have all the answers either. We can hope that one day a cure will somehow come along and end all the weary at this point. But until then, we have to trust ourselves to make the adjustments that we need in order to learn in making Crohn's easier to cope with.

Here it is, the year of 2020, and Cj is doing great! I can't say the same for this year though, because so much is happening. The COVID-19, the unrest of systemic racism, police brutality, and the flu season is about to unfold in a way where I just might be locked up at home until March rolls back around. Which is why learning about what works with your child or loved one doesn't have to be a negative impact. It can be a positive learning experience because others may need information from your experience. Just as I'm giving you my experiences I have learned on my own without any doctor's input. In the next chapter, I have written seventeen important facts I like to call my "get-it together" moments.

CHAPTER 8

Get-It Together (GIT)

My get-it together moments will guide you as a parent down this path of learning, observing, what to do, what not to do, and what to look for daily. I give these facts because it is necessary to empower yourself as I had no help with figuring some stuff out. I keep it real, and 100 percent on point at all times with what I share with you. Even if you do not use some of my knowledge, you can always adjust something I have told you to suit your child's needs as things arise. I would say you can hijack my moments to fit your child's lifestyle if needed.

It's now the year of 2020, and Cj is doing great! I can't say the same for this year though, because so much is happening. The COVID-19, the unrest of systemic racism, police brutality, and the flu season is about to unfold in a way where I just might be locked up at home until March of 2021 rolls around. I cannot afford to get the flu, COVID-19, or both. All I see is that they are both deadly and to end up with them is a death sentence, but only you might die in a matter of twenty-four hours. Okay, my imagination is in overdrive. But I can say it does sound scary for COVID and the flu to be floating around us all and at the same time. Stay healthy or make changes to become healthy.

Seventeen GIT (get-it together) moments

GIT 1. Make sure your child, family member, or friend who may have been diagnosed with Crohn's disease have a gastroenterologist specialist, as soon as you find out it's Crohn's. In the past, I have seen certain people with Crohn's be misdiagnosed, and instead of being treated for Crohn's, the person was treated as if they had an infection and was given antibiotics instead of medication for Crohn's. Ask the person's regular doctor to submit a referral to see a GI specialist. A regular health care provider/doctor will not be able to take care of the patient beyond regular checkups, physicals, and etc. However, it is best for the GI specialist to keep the regular doctor up to date with all activity.

GIT 2. It is wise to make a health binder with topics such as doctor visits (general medical), ER visits, temperature, weight loss/gain, GI specialist visits, physicals, eating habits, allergic reactions, blood draws, and medications. Keep a track of all visits to any doctor such as eye, family, health, skin, ear, or nose. This was very helpful to me as a parent because sometimes we can't remember everything due to our daily lives we are living. With having to work, maybe even attending school as I was while adding home life, I was a very busy parent including going to all medical appointments and emergency visits which will happen, depending on the condition of the child. My son had to see another GI specialist, just for us to get a second opinion.

This is also a good idea because two specialist is better than one. The binder which I had all my son's information saved, was very helpful to the second specialist. The specialist looked through it and saw that everything they wanted or needed to know about the patient was there. There was no guessing or thinking hard because all dates and times of all visits in the past was accounted for. I colored coded the binder from all topics previously discussed. Emergency room visits was red, doctor visits was green, specialist visits was blue, and etc. Keep the binder handy when going to all appointments because you can write little notes when necessary and then make changes later. The binder will become your life.

GIT 3. As previously discussed in fact number two, keeping a track of medications is the most important to me because my son's Crohn's was very difficult. The reason why I say it was difficult is because most of the medications didn't work as well. Once the specialist started him on a certain type such as Remicade, it didn't work because another medication had to be given along with Remicade. It took maybe about five months to actually tell if the meds wasn't working. I started noticing weight loss again, and it was to the point my son had to be hospitalized again. The specialist will change meds and dosages like we drink water, so it's good to have a large section in the binder just for medications. You will thank me later!

GIT 4. If possible, make appointments on the less busy days you have. I found out Mondays and Fridays were the busiest for me because it's before and after the weekend. Most people like to take care of appointments on Mondays in order to get it out the way. There are more people who will go for a Friday because they figure less people will want to handle business on a Friday and would just like to go home, but that is not the case. I would make appointments for my son on Tuesdays or Thursdays, early as possible, because if you look at society, there are few people who like to catch the worm. The times would be 8:30 a.m. or 9:00 a.m. which was best for me. I worked from 11:00 a.m. to 7:30 p.m. Monday through Friday. You will have to come up with appointments that is best suitable for you and your family.

GIT 5. With your child having Crohn's, there will be a sign for infections that may lurk due to some of the medications that will lower their immune system. I always keep a thermometer handy because a fever is one of the signs that an infection is taking place. I have seen this many, many years with my son's case because a fever that comes out of nowhere and the child isn't sick with a cold or flu, this would be a sure sign of an infection within the immune system. Report it to the specialist as soon as possible, so the child can start the antibiotics. The sooner the better!

GIT 6. Weight loss is another sign that the medication for Crohn's isn't working. This is for the child who has the symptoms of diarrhea really bad. My son had the worst case with his symptoms because everything he ate it would flow right through him. The medication that supposed to help with his Crohn's, I could tell, would stop working, and then the bathroom visits would become more frequently. Even though it sounds bad, this would be a good sign for me because I can alert the specialist early on, and let him know the meds are not working. There will be test periods when it comes to medications because some work right from the start and some don't. Some will take a few months to kick in, and some takes several months but depending on your child's system.

GIT 7. Sugar and Crohn's do not mix! Sugar can agitate the Crohn's far more than expected. There will be some things a child will still eat that may contain sugar, but limit the intake and be aware of your child's diet. Sodas and shakes are the worse for my son. If I buy sodas, it's either a 7 Up or Ginger ale for an upset stomach. My son craves the acid in sodas sometimes, so I have him mix water with it. Any way to cut sugar down in your child's diet that you can think of is a very good idea. I'm not saying that sugar is bad, I'm saying it doesn't help a Crohn's patient if they are eating it at every turn.

GIT 8. CT or MRI scans will become useful if the Crohn's patient is having problems that specialist can't resolve. If the patient is hurting in a specific area for no apparent reason and nothing is clear to the eye such as symptoms of some sort, then I would say the next step is to ask the specialist for MRI scan. This test can tell what is wrong with the patient, just as it did my son. My son was hurting for months on his left side, and he was given pain medication inside the ER. The pain meds only worked temporarily as the pain kept coming back. The pain became so unbearable that my son started crying because his back began to throb like never before. An MRI was done of his left side, and there were fistulas found in his body. A Fistula is basically a pocket of bacteria which sits in parts of the body. When the bacteria is released into the blood stream, this becomes toxic, and pain begins to affect the patient. The pain can be from an eight to a twenty on the scale. When a person has Crohn's, from my experience with my son, it seems as though the subject of pain can be more sensitive, meaning hurt more.

GIT 9. You will spend a lot of time away from work, depending on each child's case. Prepare your boss or supervisor for the information. Be truthful about everything that is going on, and I'm sure they will make things easier for you just in case you might have to take off work for long periods of time.

GIT 10. Activities and Crohn's vary for each individual. Some patients may be able to move around with no problems. There will be times where flare-ups may appear in the individual. A flare-up is where the patient starts experiencing slight pain or discomfort from disease itself. Symptoms may come back if meds held symptoms at a certain level. A flare-up can happen anytime during the course of treatment. Even if medications are working and patients begin to see a difference and seem to be better than before, a flare-up can still happen no matter how good the treatment is working.

GIT 11. New symptoms can appear, depending on each case. My son started noticing boils that would come near his rectum. At this point, there is nothing that can be done other than having the patient take Epsom salt baths during this time. The rectum becomes very sore, and sometimes, to the point where they can barely walk. If it gets this bad, purchase a cushion for them to sit on, and this can help also when they are away from home. If the child is in grade school, let all their teachers know what is going on from day one. The teachers will be able to adjust to the child's schedule especially if child has to leave for appointments. If a child has a severe case with disease and can't function properly in school, you as a parent may have to take them out of a regular school system. And sign the child up in home schooling or a school that does one class a week, such as an alternate learning facility like Cj did in eleventh grade during high school. He later enrolled back into his main high school for twelfth grade and graduated with his class.

GIT 12. Over-the-counter medications should be used with caution. If you read the fine print, most medications can become harmful to the patient's body organs, depending how much is taken. I see that these same meds can cause liver problems if not careful. This is why a specialist takes plenty of test for the patient, in order to keep up with the function of all organs while on meds for Crohn's or other problems that may arise. Anti-inflammatory meds are not good for anyone diagnosed with Crohn's. My son had to stay away from Advil, aspirin, Motrin, and Excedrin due to medication creating inflammation inside system, and this is not good for Crohn's. The only medication my son can take for pain or headaches was Tylenol. I suggest talking to your child's specialist with concerns for medications you can or can't purchase.

GIT 13. Visiting public places can be quite embarrassing for someone who is dealing with Crohn's, especially children. Children can become very irritated on the things they now have to pay more attention to. As before Crohn's, they ran around free with no worries in the world. Crohn's will definitely make you adjust and adapt to a whole new world. Standing for long periods of time is one of the problems. I say this because my son had a lot of cramping in his abdomen. Standing was not his friend. I started to think ahead as a parent, and I would let my son wait in the car if I needed to stand for long periods of time. If we had to park far away from a destination such as appointments, I would drop him off at the front door which makes it easy for him to walk in and register at the front desk for his appointments while I park the car and meet him inside the facility. When I know his appointment was nearly over, I would go get the car and meet him in the front where I dropped him off at just to keep him from walking a long distance.

GIT 14. Emergency visits will become a part of your life as the parents and the child. These types of visits can vary from person to person, depending on Crohn's and how severe it is. One minute you're sitting at home watching a movie with the family, and the next you're rushing to the ER. Yes, this can happen, and it may not be the last time. You might be at work, and you get a call from child or teacher that things are not right. Don't panic, think very calmly, and put your response into second gear, throw your sneakers on and get moving. If your child sees you're worried, that will make them worry.

So truth be told, you don't want your child to take on more than what they are already dealing with.

GIT 15. Staying overnight at other places can be easy if you plan ahead. Crohn's patients, like my son, frequently visits the bathroom more often than others, so hopefully, there are at least two bathrooms available. The timeframe inside a bathroom can be from ten minutes to forty-five minutes for my son. I notice after he eats a meal, he can feel the food passing through his stomach slowly. Sometimes, it can be painful because of the gas that form, and other times, he would be fine.

GIT 16. Sanitation and public bathrooms or public places are very important because you don't want your child to pick up any other germs or bacteria that may interfere with their Crohn's. The medications that my son takes lowers his immune system, so I make sure to stay away from others with cold or flu-like symptoms because it will be necessary. Let me just say colds and flus are not good with this disease because then the child or patient has to take antibiotics along with all meds they're already taking. From my experience with my son, taking antibiotics was just painful. I say it was painful for me to see him have nasty episodes from vomiting, to not being able to have a bowel movement. Some antibiotics can be harsh to the system and cause constipation. I would say plan ahead because this will save you a lot of wear and tear on your body as a parent. Carrying hand sanitizer and baby wipes also can only make situations like this easier and clean. The easier the visits in public, the more energy you will save for other emergencies that may pop up.

GIT 17. Comfortability for your child should be important through making adjustments from day one of diagnosis. I have learned to have an open mind and also to be creative. Trust me, you will need to learn skills as a parent as the time goes by or should I say years. As a parent, be mindful of Crohn's because what you're experiencing is far less than what your child is experiencing.

I hope this information has helped or is helping parents out there in the world because I didn't have any clue on what was going on or what to expect. Put all your skills you have learned over the years to work, and there will be days where you can relax. Until they find a cure, I say be well and enjoy the good moments when you can. This information doesn't have to only pertain to a child. If you know someone with IBD, this can help others as well. Have a blessed learning experience, and take care of yourself.

THE END

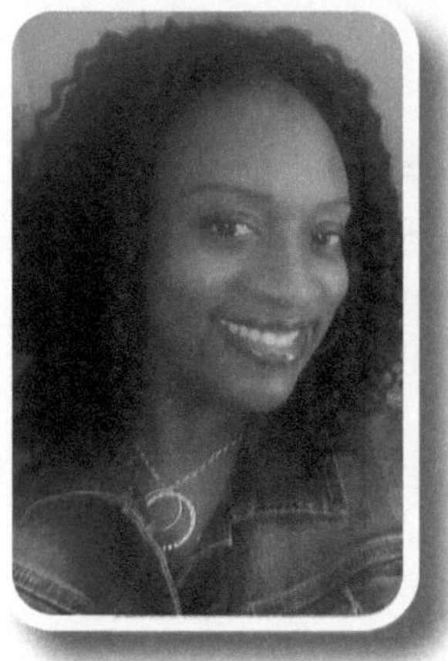

Rachel M. Cooper worked at the Veterans Affair Hospital for thirty years in Palo Alto, California, learning from experiences in the healthcare field. *Parenting a Child with Crohn's Disease* is her first book inspired by her son's trials in life.